Awakening Your Sexual Ecstasy:

The Trail of Sexuality for Lovers.

By

Fiona Perkins.

Table of Contents

Introduction

The most emotionally charged aspect of our life is sex. We carry a lot of mental expectations, fears, and emotional baggage into the bedroom every time. It makes sense why we don't always feel excited about our sexual experiences. Tantra is a spiritual concept that aims to help acquaint you with who you are and live in the present. It is fundamentally a tradition in which waking is gained by enlightenment and or meditation, and oneness is sought through closeness and love.

In the west, it has been largely followed for its emphasis on using sexual union as one of its means of awakening. Tantra is perceived as a light instrument that can be gotten easily by paying a set amount for the workshop or classes, while its profound ad holy meaning is neglected in reality, only a tiny fraction of tantra interacts with sex, and solely as a path to union with the divine.

Although this book discusses Tantra and sex, Tantra spans different facets as it conforms to the concept of sexuality, intimacy, and spirituality, You'll learn how to relax into your body and feel wonderful sensations via breathing techniques, active meditations, and erotic rituals. You'll also learn how to improve your awareness of your partner's body.

This book tends to explore only the sexual aspect and aims to correct various notions that it is only used to

answer sexual prayers instead of adopting a particular lifestyle.
In this book, you'll learn

- How tantra tends to awaken inner desire and lover
- How to actively offer and receive pleasure
- The set tantric Ideals as connected to sex and sexuality and
- Benefits of practising yoga either alone or as couples.

Chapter 1

Sex and Tantric Set Ideals

Tantra is an old Indian tradition that has been around for more than 5,000 years. Tantra translates to "knit together" in Sanskrit. Tantric sex is a technique to "weave" the material with the spiritual for those who meditate in Buddhist and Hindu traditions.

This method emphasizes the value of closeness in sexual encounters and combines sexuality and spirituality.

Tantra doesn't just focus on sexual pleasure, though.

The emphasis is primarily on enjoying your body and experiencing increased sensuality. Spirituality, sexuality, and a state of mindfulness are all incorporated into the practice. It promotes sensual enjoyment that can be had either by oneself or with a companion.

There is no greater or lower in the tantric cosmos. It encourages risk-taking and unconventional behavior. Whether it's fixing a car, sweeping the floor, or making love, the small, everyday tasks of life become extraordinary when we put our all into them.

If you want more passion in your romantic relationships, think and act passionately and you'll find that you're attracting more of it than you ever imagined. Make time and space for your body to let go if you believe that you might benefit from surrendering more in your life. Paint the picture of your life on the canvas that you have created. You'll be amazed by the impact if you apply this strategy to your sexual life.

Tantric sex aims to achieve spiritual or energetic touch while having sensuous fun. Orgasm is not always the desired outcome. It's about having a strong, enlightened connection with either your spouse or yourself. It entails movements, sounds, and breathing to stimulate sexual energy.

Tantra is not exclusively sexual activity. It's an Eastern philosophy that covers a range of spiritual ideas.

Tantric practices like yoga, meditation, and breathing can boost one's sexual arousal. The idea that tantric sex includes wild, unrestrained sexual encounters is a frequent fallacy. Tantric practices are both a mental and a spiritual discipline, though they can help you become more open to new feelings.

Another fallacy regarding tantra is the idea that a partner is always required. Tantric sex is often practiced by couples, although it can also be done alone.

Having a tantric experience doesn't even need having genital contact or sexual intercourse. In addition to practicing tantra to feel more connected to your mind and body and to give yourself pleasure, you can have sexual encounters to enrich your experience. In actuality, the main objectives of people who use tantric practices or adhere to the tantric path are soul liberation and consciousness expansion. Tantric sex is simply one method out of many that are available to do this.

Additionally, bending into difficult stances or positions is not a part of tantric sex. Being intimate with your spouse in a way that is comfortable for you is important.

You are allowed to move and touch however you and your spouse think is most comfortable.

You might try a few strategies to get ready before exploring tantric sex. Making the ideal setting is the first step. An environment that is relaxing and free from outside disturbances is ideal for practising tantric methods. It's time to unwind and settle in once you've located your favourite location.

Reflection / Meditation

This entails pausing for a moment to be mindful of your surroundings, whether you have experience with meditation or not. Make full use of your senses to take in everything around you.

In contrast to other forms of sexual union, tantric union invites you to completely enjoy every facet of your relationship, including the spiritual and holy. The most effective way to do this is through tantric meditation. When you practice meditation, you are urged to concentrate on one or more aspects of your relationship, such as a specific feeling, or to rise and fall in your level of desire.

You learn to appreciate each moment, each glance, and each touch rather than being solely preoccupied with ejaculation or orgasm. You may go toward spiritual happiness at every instant of your relationship. You take your time to increase and heighten your enjoyment and to prolong the pleasant experience.

During tantric sex, you also honor your partner by getting to know him or her better and in a more meaningful way. This enables your partner to develop in love and sexual contentment while also helping you to learn more about your partner. The highest rising in love is attainable if you keep in touch with life's wonders when you're in a relationship.

Tantra's ultimate goal is to achieve this sensation, which elevates sex to a spiritual level. If you can, always stay in touch with the divine in your mate. By putting judgments aside and looking behind the person's outward characteristics, you may do this. Look into your partner's deepest essence, touch their body with love and regard, and learn to fly together while being fueled by your beautiful connection.

Breath

Tantra practice requires us to intentionally let go of all of our preconceived notions and prejudices. You'll also need to master expectation-letting. You won't truly be having an orgasm if you're thinking about what sort of orgasm you want to have in your head.Our imaginations have the power to both restrict and generate sexual energy. Being present requires a long, ongoing process of exploration. One of the easiest methods to quiet racing

thoughts and center yourself is to control your breathing.
Tantra practice requires us to intentionally let go of all of our preconceived notions and prejudices. You'll also need to master expectation-letting. You won't truly be having an orgasm if you're thinking about what sort of orgasm you want to have in your head.
Our imaginations have the power to both restrict and generate sexual energy. Being present requires a long, ongoing process of exploration. One of the easiest methods to quiet racing thoughts and center yourself is to control your breathing
Take a steady, deep breath in, then let it out slowly to empty your lungs.

Until you find the rhythm, keep doing this.

The objective of tantric breathing is to inhale deeply enough to cause sensation to begin in your genital organs.

Movement

Relax while lying flat on your back. Arc your back and elevate your pelvis as you breathe. Repeating this will help you establish a rhythm, feel yourself letting go of stress, and begin to connect with your body and emotions.

Tantric practices encourage intimate, close touch and let you and your partner feel free to feel one other's bodies. Couples can learn what they truly enjoy while also imparting knowledge to their companion.

Tantric sessions can last for several hours and are intended to be fulfilling. To appreciate intimacy and closeness for as long as possible, many people try to delay climax.

If you and your partner are prepared to experiment with tantric sex, you should start by practicing eye contact. Face your companion, put on your clothes, and look each other in the eyes. Develop your breathing methods, and time your breaths. Tantric methods can be incorporated once you've established a rhythm.

Once you are undressed, you can start touching, sensing, and moving with your partner in the ways that feel right to you. Maintaining eye contact and concentrating on your breathing is crucial in this situation. Being in the moment and savoring each sensation is all that matters.

The female represents every woman in the universe during tantric sex. A spontaneous display of devotional worship is how the man shows his love and trust. The woman consequently spreads open like a lotus flower, radiating tranquillity, beauty, and joy. In return, the male yields, letting go of his ego as he

becomes submerged in the totality of his partner's feminine strength.
Every man in the world is represented by the male companion, who seems to his loved one as an all-powerful deity. She yields to his ardour, lust, and vitality. She embraces her lover without resistance, realising her inner strength as she lets go. When you feel free to completely abandon your divine feminine and male identities, the moments you spend together are the most beautiful and sensual.

Chapter 2

Your Inner Desires Being Awakened.

You can develop into your own best lover through tantra. Tantra can be practised in a relationship. Solo Tantra is as significant, though. It's the ideal starting point. The most fulfilling thing you can do is have a close, sensual relationship with yourself.

Start by focusing on your own eyes. Look into your non-dominant eye intently in a mirror.

Now, discuss something positive about yourself or something you have forgiven yourself for. At first, this will certainly seem unusual, but developing this kind of self-rapport is crucial.

This is a powerful, deep healing that can help you rebalance and awaken your inner love. There is an unending reservoir of love that is continuously burning inside of you. Discover the hidden worlds and sacred temple of your heart through mystical journeying. Receive positive reprogramming as you immerse yourself in the healing powers of unwavering love. As you continue your path, you will eventually encounter the greatest love within.

It's time to take yourself on a Tantric date once you've started developing a rapport with yourself. Consider treating yourself to a fancy dinner and giving yourself plenty of time to appreciate each flavour on your plate. Then, to stimulate your senses, watch a steamy movie or attend a burlesque performance. Visit your neighborhood sex shop to select a new toy or flavor of lubricant to cap off the adventure. Make love to yourself after returning home and enjoying a sumptuous dinner and a hot bath.

Now is the ideal time to try something new. What arouses you the most? Different sensual languages titillate us all differently. Some of us need sound, while others need sight. And for some individuals, contact is the primary stimulant. Or act out a spicy short narrative while giving yourself an erotic massage. Tantric dates don't usually entail having sexual contact. They focus more on arousing erotic energy.

These opportunities are also fantastic for playing with new toys and trying on new personas. You might wish to employ nipple clamps if you believe you have an inner dominatrix. You can also feel like experimenting with an alternative gender presentation.

You can explore with Solo Tantra. You won't have to defend yourself to anyone and can immerse yourself entirely in your sensual universe.

Tantra emphasizes physical and mental development because the mind is the primary source of all sensual experiences. Spending time alone in thought, free from the demands to interact with people, is essential if you truly realize that you are the creator of your world and are living your life as you go through it. Discovering your body's functions and sensations is crucial, likewise providing it with the necessary physical care. Whether its a long shower or a challenging workout, make time and space for activities that calm your mind and awaken your body.

Never stop engaging in masturbation. It's a growing practice where you can learn what you like and obtain the healing you need for any sex-related trauma or shame you may have. It essentially consists of developing a close bond with oneself because it is the foundation for developing close bonds with others. Regular alone time is the ideal setting for indulging in self-pleasuring. The best approach to learning more about what makes you physically on or off is to do this. Tantra promotes and praises self-pleasuring as a means of sensitising your own body and increasing your receptivity to receiving and imparting pleasure. The more you respect your amazing body, the more capable it will be of receiving the respect you would like from others. Instead of waiting for someone else to "do it" for you, it's critical to consistently fuel and stimulates your own body. Sometimes we are discouraged for several reasons, such as guilt for taking time for ourselves, emotions of shame, or embarrassment.

You must let rid of whatever holds you back. Both yourself and a lover should give you the time and consideration you deserve. To feel secure enough to allow another person to artistically and sensually satisfy you, you must be aware of your own body and what makes you feel good.

Spend some time discovering and getting to know your own body. You can get started by completing the exercises below.

Tantra urges you to awaken all facets of your sexuality to fully enjoy a full and abundant existence. Self-indulgence and sharing time in meditation with your lover are two ways to ignite your sexual energy.

Any form of sexually stimulating physical activity can also awaken your sexuality. You can feel energised by dancing to help you remember what it's like to be fully present with love and respect for yourself. Your senses of hearing, touch, and sight are stimulated as well as your sex drives through simple sexual movements.

- Start dancing to some sexy music. Begin moving as though you were dancing for a lover who was observing you.

- Visualise the person you want to stand in for your "partner" in your imagination. It could be a real or imaginary partner.

- Start gently and sensually taking off your clothes. Show your devoted sweetheart more and more of yourself over time.

Every part of your body is enamoured by him or her.

- When you're completely naked, dance vigorously while savouring your attractiveness. Liberate your hips and let them swing in all their joy. Allow the powerful sexual energy to flare up like a fire. As the energy rises your centre channel moves your spine in a circular motion.

- After the dancing is complete, lie down and picture your partner gently blowing a warm breath over your body.

Imagine your lover's hands caressing you with desire as you stroke your body.

Let your enthusiasm grow without keeping anything back. Try touching your face, hair, and other untouched parts of your body. Lovely stroke your genitalia.

Let your imagined lover's hands carry you to a state of orgasmic pleasure. Take a peaceful nap after the dramatic waves have subsided.It’s normal to desire to be held, caressed, and cherished.Everybody requires and wants contact, yet many individuals spend a lot of their life devoid of soothing touch. Sometimes men and women go hunting for sex only so that they may feel physically linked to another human being.

Keep exploring methods to open up and receive more personal contact.

Start by touching yourself, and discovering which strokes and pressures are sexiest and most pleasant. Later, this is valuable knowledge to bring to lovemaking. Informed, mindful touch is a master key in opening to the universal spirit of love.

Chapter 3

The Skills to Heighten Intimacy

Without conscious effort, intimacy can plateau and a partnership with another person can start to feel more like a routine than a conscious choice. Although it applies to all of our relationships, the effects are strong in romantic and sexual dynamics. To cultivate intimacy, one must invest time, effort, and commitment. Active communication is one of our most effective methods for building relationships. You have the power to change your relationships exactly how you want them to be and keep fostering greater intimacy with your partner(s).

Set Aside Time For Profound Conversations

Deep discussions can promote emotional closeness. Stop worrying about the stress at work or on your to-do list. At the end of the day, express your feelings. When your speaking partner is speaking, try not to constantly judge or evaluate them. Pay attention. Vulnerability is necessary for establishing a close bond, and it can be simple to succumb to the urge to exert control over a situation when having difficult conversations.

When our love feels urgent, our brains frequently default to an all-or-nothing response. Rather than sorting through the murky complexity of a situation, we seek certainty. In these circumstances, embrace curiosity rather than control. Ask your partner(s) more questions when your brain wants to assume the worst, give them a chance to clarify, and give them room to grow as a person. Moments of growth and understanding like these have the potential to strengthen your intimate bond because they will teach you more about one another.

Make sex a top priority.

Sex often takes a very low priority in relationships. Prioritize and uphold physical connection and intimacy. Additionally, over time, sexual needs may alter. As a result, alter your routine and try something new. To maintain a healthy and exciting sex life, you can experiment with new sex positions or locations.

Instead of jumping right into sex after getting ready, give yourself some time to warm up. You could meditate or alternately shake various body parts with one another. Massages for one another are a great idea as well. It's important to let go, connect, and enjoy yourself.

You're in tune with each other and with yourself now. You're ready for the ritual to start because the scene is

set.Tantric sex may seem frightening to you if you've studied the Kama Sutra. Most of us lack the flexibility necessary to contort ourselves into sexy yoga poses.
However, the focus of Tantra is not on physical prowess. How conscious and in the moment you are while making love is much more crucial. Depending on how you focus your energies and tune in to your partner's body, you could have sex in the same position every day and still feel completely different.

What then can help you and your partner stay awake during sex? Start by developing your giving and receiving skills. Face each other as you sit down. Pose a leg-crossing. Starting at the top of the skull and moving downward, alternately stroke each other's bodies.

Putting your feet behind your partner's back while sitting on his lap is another beneficial exercise. In particular, when you begin to breathe at the same rate and feel your body moving as a unit, this is a very intimate position for connecting. This is a fantastic position for dildo or penis penetration as well.

Whatever position you select, it should encourage the flow of sexual energy within and between your bodies. Your genitalia, breasts, eyes, hands, and tongue are the most crucial points of contact. Remember that penetration isn't the primary goal of sex and be inventive in how you generate sexual energy.

To titillate your partner, use your mouth, tongue, and breath. Tease them by brushing a feather across them. Make sure to alternate between quick, harsh touches and soft, gradual ones. Although you very well may come, that is not the objective. Don't bring any subliminal requests for your partner or expectations into the ritual.

Tantric philosophy has a concept known as "three strokes for 30." In other words, it's preferable to have three deliciously precise, expertly applied touches rather than 30 sloppy ones. Giving your partner those "three touches" with all of your body and mind is essential in a loving relationship because the focus is everything.

Finally, make an effort to intentionally enjoy the afterglow of your recent sexual experience, either by yourself or with your partner. Your body will continue to experience the energy for several days.

Dance-Based Communication

Dancing fosters sexual connection and functions as a powerful treatment for relationship problems that have not been handled. Dance is a nonverbal means for lovers to express their affection for one another. Due to its inherent sensuality, it releases mood-enhancing brain chemicals that permeate the entire body through the circulatory system. The mind loses control when the body moves voluntarily, opening a channel of communication that is not limited to language.

The kundalini energy, potent sexual energy that rises from the back of the sacrum, can also be awakened by dancing. When you dance, the energy from the song can shimmer its way up your spine, energising your chakras and activating the head chakra, resulting in an increased level of awareness.

Kundalini energy will be inactive if your hips are stiff and your sacrum is tightly grasped. Dancing helps you move your hips more independently from the rest of your body, which allows them to express their personalities and causes your kundalini energy to uncurl and begin to ascend.

Loosening your pelvis will also make both of you more physically flexible during passionate acts. A man will also discover that he has improved control over ejaculation.

You can enroll in a variety of dance classes, from salsa to ballroom dancing, to learn how to move your pelvis, but if you are first a bit self-conscious, you can practice in private at home. Play some fantastic music loudly, then start moving

Wild Imaginations

Imagination is an aspect of your unconscious mind, and it plays a fundamental role in relationships. A large part of sexual attraction arises through a kind of creative process within the lover, meaning that what goes on in your mind is often more important than what is true of your beloved. Because of this, we can project any fantasy onto our interactions with our partners. This facility, unique to humans, can be used to great advantage in erotic play and sex games.

Think of your imagination as a muscle that you can either use regularly or let atrophy through neglect. We envision our life into reality. Because we are who we think we are. We could analyse this concept further The beauty of fantasising is that its personal. It's your private world that you can manifest into reality if you choose.
Experiencing that niche with an affectionate partner helps keep the flames of passion and intimacy in the

relationship. Sharing good memories together is a pleasant way to gaining sexual freedom with your partner.You may believe you are not in the mood for sex, especially after a hectic, stressful day, but you still want to spend time with your spouse; play may offer you this, and who knows where it can go. Imaginative play may let you leave adult obligations behind, and leave the route clean for intimacy.

Laughing also boosts circulation in your body–not to mention attraction, desire, and playful sexiness.

Think of life as a game sometimes, and you'll find your relationship becomes more sensual, intimate, and enjoyable.

Chapter 4

Infusing Trust

It's crucial to accept and celebrate each other's differences if you want to awaken and ignite. Your differences are what ignite the sexual passion and excitement that can lead to orgasmic fulfillment. Embrace your partner's power and masculinity, ladies. Love your partner's sensuous side, men. Spend time away from obligations, pay attention to various forms of contact, and communicate with each other in different ways if you have forgotten what initially attracted and sexy about each other. Letting tantra guide you will help you rediscover the qualities that you formerly found so alluring.

Keep in mind that your partnership is holy as you learn more about tantra. Your love is a gift that should be revered and respected. As you explore the fresh ground, be kind to one another. Try new things, and learn what your spouse likes and dislikes by listening to him or her.

You'll both start to slow down and spend time getting to know each other again during your tantric trip, which is one thing you'll notice. Tantric meditation techniques are straightforward, yet the life-altering impacts they have can give long-lasting or even waning romances fresh vitality.

Tantra might help you find new ways to enjoy your time together, even if your relationship is going well.

Learn what works for you both as an emotional and sexual partnership as you experiment with different meditation techniques while listening to your spouse. Find traditions that you appreciate and can teach you. Recognize and accept your many urges, feelings, and emotions, and allow them to be fully present during sex and other relationship-related activities.

To engage in solo and intimate Tantric sex, we must first create a holy and secure environment for ourselves. Even while you don't need to wait for the ideal surroundings to practice tantra, a peaceful, lovely setting can enable you to establish an atmosphere that is suitable for meditation. You may make a mystical, sacred sanctuary isolated from the outside world by paying close attention to the little things. It's simpler to focus on your spouse and to make each other happy and comfortable when you're both in your place.

The ideal situation would be for you to commit an entire room to your tantric practice, but even a small area like a bedroom may be quite effective.You will be able to create a tranquil retreat where you may retreat and enjoy your time together by making a well-considered choice of colors, materials, and ritual items. It is worthwhile to spend in the aesthetic ambiance of your area. You will want to spend time in your place if it is inviting to enter and feels comfortable.

If you don't have enough space in your house to set up a dedicated tantra area, you can still make the most of what you currently have by adding objects that you solely use for meditation. You can alter the atmosphere of your room with a particular bedspread, lovely candles, a yantra, or a wall hanging featuring tantric devotion.

Lovemaking takes on a sacred quality thanks to tantric rituals and meditation. You should be interacting with your companion in a peaceful, harmonious setting.

Both of you will feel more at ease and focused as a result of this. You will feel more sensuous and alive if you surround yourself with lovely things.

A tantric meditation on its own is giving your spouse a good time. The purpose of oral sex is to encourage you and your partner to live in the now and harmony with one another. Oral gratification is a fairly solitary practice that allows you to concentrate entirely on your partner's reactions while giving one specific area of their body your undivided attention. Oral allows you to focus entirely on the moment and the exquisite enjoyment of your partner, unlike any other sex act.

This is a great chance to learn more and let go of any of your preconceived views if you have any kind of apprehension regarding oral sex. Tantra urges you to see and appreciate the beauty in every aspect of the human form, including the genitalia, seeing it as a manifestation of the divine. Take a hot shower together to start these meditations, and feel eager to do something sensual and intensely enjoyable. Jump in and have fun, keeping in mind that tantra is also referred to as the great Experiment.

The harmony that may exist between the masculine and feminine principles is best exemplified through mutual oral gratification. A pair may have a fulfilling feeling of balance as a result of giving and receiving in equal measure, much like Shiva and Shakti did. You and your partner will grasp what arouses and fills you with joy as you give each other more pleasure. An important aspect of tantric practice is oral gratification, which may help you master your partner's physical cravings. You can discover over time that oral gratification is hotter and perhaps more personal than sexual activity.

Chapter 5

Achieving Orgasm

The truth is that there is very little agreement on what constitutes an orgasm. Most of us imagine an orgasm to be a climax that occurs during genital stimulation. Typically, those encounters are brief and intense. Even while they can be exhilarating, orgasms are much more than just these passionate volcanic outbursts.

What does orgasm signify in a deeper sense? It is described as a letting go of stress and a submission to the energy that flows through our body. Many events can be seen as orgasmic when one is in this mindset. Consider a time when you cried so much that you felt as though a terrible storm had passed or when your body shook with unrestrained laughter.

The tantric method to sex enables you to access orgasmic energy, the most potent healing force available to us as human beings, at all times throughout sex. All you need to do is open up and connect to the ever-flowing source to experience the perpetual orgasm that the cosmos is in. A full-body, cosmic orgasm can be experienced by both men and women. The nectar of true sexual fulfillment is your birthright, but frequently we fool ourselves for a short fix, an instant orgasm, and an instant ejaculation. You can view climax as a path to transcendence and, ultimately, as a profound source of healing and renewal as you reframe your expectations of what sex should look and feel like. When practicing tantric meditation, allow yourself to follow the natural flow of energy and emotion between your bodies without trying to control the results. Without effort, strategy, or plan of action, a tantric orgasm occurs. Your bodies expand smoothly as you enter a level of oneness where you can enjoy completely intimate pleasure while still being alert and conscious.

Men's Orgasmic Nature

Ejaculation is typically associated with orgasm in men, however, it is a minor physiologic function in comparison to the stunning, full-body orgasm attainable during tantric sex. A man can have the ability to use his orgasmic energy to fill his entire body with repetition. He can enjoy hours of sexual bliss without ejaculating. He can learn to climax like a woman by channeling his sex energy upward and outward like an ecstatic cosmic geyser.

Women’s Orgasmic Nature

It's critical for both partners to realize that penetration by itself won't cause a woman to orgasm. Since most women require clitoris stimulation to climax, this should always take place during your union. You can also stimulate erogenous regions like the nipples, breasts, neck, and other places that your spouse finds attractive to increase orgasm. The nipples are a particularly good area to touch because the clitoris and the nipples' nerves are directly connected. Both the inner and exterior of the yoni engorge and swell during the preparation for orgasm. The yoni secretes fluids, and the woman may feel an inside aching or a physical want for penetration. Nipples become erect, and blood pressure, pulse rate, and breathing rate all rise. The woman will be able to plunge into the enormous ocean of orgasm and ride the waves of euphoric joy if she is calm, flowing with her energy and emotions, and able to let go of control

Ejaculating Under Control

Try one or more of these techniques to keep the semen if you feel like you might ejaculate during sex. Although mastering these techniques can take some time, give your body the time it needs to adjust to the new ways of moving sexual energy.

Some of the techniques can be helped with by your partner.

- Unwind and stop thinking about your genitalia.

Imagine the orgasmic energy in your body rising through your body.
Imagine your sexual energy rising and flowing toward your heart as you inhale. Release it into your partner's heart when you exhale, from your heart chakra.

- Maintaining your genitals inside your partner, assume the Yab Yum position. Together, breathe and sway, maintaining your intimate proximity while allowing

the energy dip that helps you unwind and prolong arousal.

- Hold your pressure until you no longer feel the urge to ejaculate on the point just below your glands. firmly press into the perineum's indentation.

- Gently rub your testicles, then move your fingers along your thighs, up your belly, and then toward your heart.

The results are dramatic . Anything from peacefulness and feeling tingly to developing a deep sense of catharsis or even seeing visions.

The secret is to let go of your expectations and fully commit to the exercise. When you expand your definition of orgasms, you'll find erotic possibilities everywhere.

Chapter 6

Attaining Sexual Satisfaction

Simple actions like breathing, kissing, and massage can all provide intensely pleasurable mystical experiences. To get there, you must fully inhabit your body, remain in tune with your partner, and immerse yourselves in each sexual moment while letting everything else fade away.

Breath is regarded in tantra as the entrance to the divine. When you breathe deliberately, energy will follow the path of that breath and leave behind new energy. Your senses will become more acute as you replenish your energy and vigor, and you'll be more receptive to experiencing divine joy.

You will learn more about your body as you become more conscious of your breathing and how it affects you. You'll unwind more, bringing greater creativity and self-assurance to every situation. Use your breath to relax if you're under pressure. Make time each day to go outside, walk, breathe in the clean air, and exhale the stagnant air. Particularly during sex, you will have easier access to subtle energy realms.

Sex and Breath

Tantra promotes deep breathing to stimulate all of the body's regions. Every cell in your body is revitalized by the fresh oxygen you inhale, which makes you feel lively and invigorated. This is the first step toward having a full-body orgasm, in which your entire body—not just your genitalia—comes to life with sensation and delightful emotions. Deep breathing helps the emotions of pleasure you experience during massage, foreplay, and intercourse spread throughout your entire body. You'll limit your enjoyment and emotional release if you hold your breath. More enjoyable feelings will circulate throughout your body as you breathe more.

Numerous tantric meditations include partner breathing, which can help harmonise your two selves. It aids in your relaxation and helps you focus on one another.

Another effective strategy for fostering sex compatibility between lovers is a kiss. The more you kiss each other, the more likely it is that you will feel at ease with one another. Additionally, you are more likely to be aware of how your partner is feeling and to intuitively understand the kind of physical contact that person wants at that precise time. Of course, a fantastic kiss is an ideal method to set the stage for great sex between the two of you.

The Tantric Embrace

The holy sexual connection of lovers is mirrored in kissing. It may involve intense sexual activity. The penetrating tongue and sensual giving of the lips evoke the yoni's softness and the lingam's penetration, respectively. Kissing has a significant place in tantric sex. The act of kissing ignites passion by sending sensual messages throughout the entire body. A satisfying kiss can arouse your

senses and is essential for getting you ready for tantric meditation and sex. The focus and consciousness you bring to the tantric kiss determine whether it is delicate and tender or passionate and animalistic. Be conscious of how you kiss and how it makes you feel to be kissed.
Your sensitivity to other aspects of making love will grow as a result.

Try out a few of these sensual massage techniques to see which ones you enjoy giving and which ones your partner enjoys receiving. Make sure you respect your partner's entire body. Don't only concentrate on the erogenous areas that will thrill them. To foster a strong sense of trust, let your spouse unwind and enjoy the massage.

Flowing

Using the entire hand or just the tips, create lengthy, sensual strokes. Use a lot of oil to ensure smooth movement.

Kneading

Is the rhythmic squeezing and releasing of large areas of skin with both hands. Apply this to the body's fleshier regions, including the thighs, belly, hips, and buttocks.

Thumbing circles

Circling with your thumbs in small, deep motions. This stroke, especially on fleshier parts of the body, is excellent for releasing any tension held in the muscles when applied with pressure.

Feathering

Use your fingertips to apply light strokes. The skin tingles as a result of this delicate stroke, which activates the sensory nerves in the skin.

You need to be completely focused on each other to develop an explosive sexual connection.

Tantric sex can last for an hour or be prolonged for several days! Really, it depends on you and your companion.

Start by indulging in a few hours of tantric sexual encounters. Once you've made a connection between each other in a domain outside of the physical plane, you'll quickly come to the conclusion that two hours of sex is simply not enough.

www.ingramcontent.com/pod-product-compliance
Lightning Source LLC
LaVergne TN
LVHW052056160826
845678LV00015B/3264
9798358621626